BLOOD TYPE A

COOKBOOK AND FOOD LIST GUIDE

Nutritional Diet recipes with a 28-day Meal plan to Ignite your energy and transform your wellbeing

Dr. ANDY PALMER

TABLE OF CONTENTS

4

Chapter 1

Introduction

Understanding Blood Type A

Blood Type A individuals are characterized by specific genetic markers on their red blood cells. These markers, known as antigens, influence various aspects of health and wellness. People with Blood Type A are believed to have certain physiological traits and predispositions that can be addressed through a tailored diet. Individuals with Blood Type A are often described as having a sensitive immune system and a well-functioning digestive system. They may be more susceptible to stress-related conditions and benefit from practices that promote relaxation and balance.

The recommended diet for Blood Type A is designed to support these unique characteristics. Typically, it involves a plant-based approach with an emphasis on fresh, organic produce. Foods like vegetables, fruits, legumes, and lean proteins are encouraged, while dairy and certain animal products may be limited.

Understanding the intricacies of Blood Type A lays the foundation for a personalized and holistic approach to health. By aligning dietary choices with the specific needs of this blood type, individuals may experience improved energy levels, weight management, and overall well-being.

The science behind Blood Type A

The science behind Blood Type A centers on the presence of specific antigens on the surface of red blood cells. Individuals with

Blood Type A carry the A antigen, a protein that triggers distinct immune responses. This genetic distinction is a result of inherited genes from both parents.

Scientifically, Blood Type A is associated with a well-functioning digestive system and heightened immune sensitivity. It is believed that these genetic factors influence how the body responds to certain foods, affecting overall health. For instance, Blood Type A individuals may exhibit greater resilience to certain infections but may also be more prone to stress-related conditions. Research suggests that tailoring dietary choices to align with the unique characteristics of Blood Type A can yield health benefits. A plant-based diet rich in fresh, organic produce is often recommended, emphasizing a balance of nutrient-dense foods. Understanding the genetic underpinnings of Blood Type A provides a foundation for crafting dietary strategies that promote optimal well-being and may contribute to a healthier, more harmonious lifestyle.

Importance of Tailored Nutrition

Tailored nutrition for individuals with Blood Type A is paramount for optimizing health and well-being. The unique genetic markers and characteristics associated with Blood Type A suggest that a personalized approach to diet can have a significant impact on overall health outcomes.

One key aspect is the potential influence on the immune system. Blood Type A individuals may possess a more sensitive immune response, making it crucial to select foods that support immune resilience. Tailoring the diet to include immune-boosting nutrients can enhance the body's ability to ward off infections and maintain optimal health.

Furthermore, the digestive system of Blood Type A individuals is believed to function optimally under specific dietary conditions. Adopting a diet rich in plant-based foods, including fruits, vegetables, and legumes, aligns with the genetic predispositions associated with Blood Type A. This not only supports digestive health but may also contribute to improved nutrient absorption and energy metabolism.

Chapter 2

Blood Type A Basics

Characteristics of Blood Type A

Blood Type A individuals are characterized by distinct traits that influence both their physical and physiological well-being. These individuals typically exhibit a heightened sensitivity in their immune system, making them more attuned to environmental and dietary factors. This heightened immune response may contribute to their resilience against certain infections but could also render them more susceptible to stress-related conditions.

In terms of personality, Blood Type A individuals are often described as cooperative, detail-oriented, and organized. They tend to thrive in structured environments and may experience increased stress levels when faced with disorganization or uncertainty.

Physiologically, those with Blood Type A often have a well-functioning digestive system. This characteristic suggests that their bodies may efficiently metabolize and process certain types of foods. As a result, a diet tailored to their genetic predispositions, such as a plant-based and balanced nutritional approach, is often recommended to promote optimal health.

Health Implications

The Blood Type A classification carries specific health implications that guide lifestyle choices for individuals with this blood type. One significant aspect is the association with a well-functioning immune system. Blood Type A individuals may demonstrate resilience to certain infections, showcasing an immune system that efficiently responds to external threats.

However, this heightened immune sensitivity can also present challenges, potentially making Blood Type A individuals more prone to stress-related conditions. Managing stress becomes crucial to maintaining overall well-being, as these individuals may experience greater physiological responses to stressful situations.

From a dietary perspective, understanding the health implications of Blood Type A informs the selection of foods that complement its genetic characteristics. A diet rich in plant-based foods is often recommended to support digestive health and mitigate potential health risks associated with this blood type.

Benefits of Blood Type A Diet

The Blood Type A diet offers a range of health benefits tailored to the unique genetic characteristics of individuals with this blood type.

1. **Immune System Support:** The diet aligns with the immune system sensitivity often associated with Blood Type A, providing nutrients that support a robust immune response.

2. **Digestive Harmony:** Blood Type A individuals typically have a well-functioning digestive system. The diet emphasizes plant-based foods, promoting digestive health and efficient nutrient absorption.

3. **Weight Management:** Following the recommended diet for Blood Type A may contribute to effective weight management. The emphasis on

whole, nutrient-dense foods can help regulate metabolism and support a healthy weight.

4. **Stress Reduction:** Blood Type A individuals may be more prone to stress-related conditions. The diet includes foods and nutrients believed to help manage stress, fostering overall emotional well-being.

5. **Energy Optimization:** Tailoring nutrition to the specific needs of Blood Type A can enhance energy levels. The diet encourages the consumption of foods that align with the genetic characteristics, promoting sustained vitality throughout the day.

6. **Balanced Lifestyle:** Adopting a Blood Type A-friendly diet goes beyond individual meals; it encourages a

holistic approach to health, encompassing lifestyle choices that complement genetic predispositions.

Chapter 3

Getting Started with Blood Type A Diet

Creating a Blood Type A-Friendly Kitchen

Designing a kitchen that caters to the specific dietary needs of Blood Type A individuals involves thoughtful choices and organization.

Here's a guide to creating a Blood Type A-friendly kitchen:

1. **Plant-Centric Pantry:** Stock your pantry with a variety of whole, plant-based foods. Include grains like quinoa and brown rice, legumes such as lentils and chickpeas, and a diverse selection of fruits and vegetables.

2. **Organic Options:** Prioritize organic produce to minimize exposure to

pesticides and additives. Opt for organic fruits, vegetables, and grains whenever possible to align with the Blood Type A diet recommendations.

3. **Lean Protein Sources:** Include lean protein sources suitable for Blood Type A, such as tofu, tempeh, and fish. Maintain a well-balanced selection to support the genetic characteristics associated with this blood type.

4. **Healthy Fats:** Incorporate heart-healthy fats like olive oil and avocados. These not only add flavor to meals but also provide essential nutrients for overall well-being.

5. **Herbs and Spices:** Enhance flavor without relying on excessive salt or additives by incorporating a variety of herbs and spices. Fresh herbs like

basil, cilantro, and mint can elevate the taste of Blood Type A-friendly dishes.

6. **Blood Type A Snacks:** Have convenient, Blood Type A-approved snacks readily available. This may include raw nuts, seeds, and cut-up vegetables for quick and nutritious options between meals.

7. **Limited Dairy Products:** As the Blood Type A diet often suggests limited dairy, consider alternative options like almond or soy milk for cooking and baking.

8. **Food Storage Solutions:** Organize your refrigerator and pantry to easily access Blood Type A-approved items. Labeling shelves or containers can help maintain order and simplify meal preparation.

9. **Cookware Choices:** Invest in quality cookware to prepare nutrient-rich meals. Non-stick pans, stainless steel pots, and steaming equipment can facilitate the preparation of Blood Type A-friendly recipes.

10. **Meal Planning Tools:** Utilize meal planning tools, such as a weekly calendar and shopping list, to streamline grocery shopping and ensure that your kitchen remains well-stocked with Blood Type A-compliant ingredients.

Shopping Tips for Blood Type A Diet Success

Navigating the grocery store with the specific dietary needs of Blood Type A in mind requires strategic planning. Here are some shopping tips to ensure a successful and health-focused shopping experience:

1. Plan Ahead: Before heading to the store, create a weekly meal plan based on Blood Type A dietary recommendations. This helps streamline your shopping list and prevents impulse purchases.

2. Stick to the Perimeter: Focus on the perimeter of the store where fresh produce, lean proteins, and whole foods are typically located. This minimizes exposure to processed and non-compliant foods found in the central aisles.

3. Emphasize Fresh Produce: Load your cart with a colorful array of fresh fruits and vegetables. Opt for organic options whenever possible to align with the Blood Type A diet's emphasis on clean, pesticide-free choices.

4. Lean Proteins: Choose lean protein sources suitable for Blood Type A, such as tofu, tempeh, turkey, and certain types of fish. Select fresh, unprocessed options to avoid additives.

5. Whole Grains: Incorporate whole grains like quinoa, brown rice, and oats into your shopping list. These provide fiber and essential nutrients while adhering to the Blood Type A dietary guidelines.

6. Plant-Based Options: Explore plant-based alternatives for dairy, such as almond or soy milk. Consider non-dairy yogurts and cheeses that align with Blood Type A recommendations.

7. Nuts and Seeds: Include a variety of nuts and seeds in your shopping list for

snacking or adding to meals. These nutrient-dense options offer a satisfying crunch and contribute to the Blood Type A-friendly diet.

8. Herbs and Spices: Enhance the flavor of your meals with a diverse selection of herbs and spices. Fresh options, like basil and cilantro, can be a flavorful addition to Blood Type A-approved recipes.

9. Read Labels: Be vigilant about reading product labels to identify any additives, preservatives, or non-compliant ingredients. Choose items with minimal processing and recognizable, whole-food ingredients.

10. Limit Processed Foods: Minimize the purchase of processed and

packaged foods, as these often contain additives and ingredients that may not align with the Blood Type A diet principles.

11. Stay Hydrated: Include hydrating beverages like herbal teas and water in your shopping list. Adequate hydration is essential for overall health and complements the Blood Type A lifestyle.

Chapter 4

Blood Type A Food List

Blood Type A Food List to Eat

The Blood Type A diet emphasizes a plant-based approach, with a focus on fresh, whole foods that align with the genetic characteristics associated with this blood type.

Below is a list of foods suitable for individuals with Blood Type A:

Proteins:

1. Tofu

2. Tempeh

3. Miso

4. Lentils

5. Garbanzo beans (Chickpeas)

6. Navy beans

7. Black-eyed peas

8. Turkey (lean cuts)

9. Trout

10. Salmon

Vegetables:

1. Spinach

2. Kale

3. Broccoli

4. Brussels sprouts

5. Carrots

6. Sweet potatoes

7. Collard greens

8. Swiss chard

9. Beetroot

10. Cabbage

Fruits:

1. Berries (blueberries, strawberries, raspberries)

2. Pineapple

3. Cherries

4. Apples

5. Plums

6. Papaya

7. Fig

8. Grapes

9. Watermelon

Grains:

1. Quinoa

2. Brown rice

3. Oats

4. Buckwheat

5. Millet

6. Amaranth

7. Spelt

8. Barley

9. Farro

10. Rice cakes (in moderation)

Nuts and Seeds:

1. Almonds

2. Walnuts

3. Flaxseeds

4. Chia seeds

5. Sunflower seeds

6. Pumpkin seeds

7. Pine nuts

8. Sesame seeds

9. Hazelnuts

10. Pecans

Dairy Alternatives:

1.   Almond milk

2. Soy milk

3. Rice milk

4. Goat cheese (in moderation)

5. Feta cheese (in moderation)

Herbs and Spices:

1.   Turmeric

2. Basil

3. Cilantro

4. Ginger

5. Parsley

Healthy Fats:

1.   Olive oil

2. Avocado

3. Flaxseed oil

4. Walnut oil

5. Coconut oil (in moderation)

Beverages:

1. Green tea

2. Herbal teas (peppermint, chamomile)

3. Water

4. Fresh vegetable juices (carrot, beet, spinach)

5. Cranberry juice (in moderation)

Miscellaneous:

1. Agar-agar (vegetarian gelatin)

2. Honey (in moderation)

3. Maple syrup (in moderation)

4. Tamari sauce

5. Dark chocolate (in moderation, preferably with high cocoa content)

Blood Type A Food List to Avoid or Limit

Here is a list of foods to be cautious about if you have Blood Type A:

Meats and Proteins:

1. Beef

2. Pork

3. Chicken

4. Shellfish

5. Bacon

6. Ham

7. Venison

8. Duck

9. Goose

10. Lamb

Dairy:

1. Cow's milk

2. Whole milk

3. American cheese

4. Blue cheese

5. Brie

6. Camembert

7. Ice cream

8. Buttermilk

9. Cottage cheese

10. Parmesan cheese

Grains:

1. Wheat

2. White flour

3. Rye

4. Corn

5. Barley

6. Buckwheat

7. Bulgar

8. Granola

9. Wheat germ

10. Couscous

Vegetables:

1. Tomatoes

2. Eggplant

3. Potatoes (white and sweet)

4. Bell peppers

5. Corn

6. Lima beans

7. Avocado

8. Olives

9. Artichokes

10. Radishes

Nuts and Seeds:

1. Cashews

2. Pistachios

3. Peanuts

4. Pumpkin seeds

5. Sunflower seeds

Oils:

1. Cottonseed oil

2. Peanut oil

3. Sesame oil

4. Corn oil

5. Canola oil

Sweeteners:

1. White sugar

2. Brown sugar

3. Corn syrup

4. High fructose corn syrup

5. Artificial sweeteners

Beverages:

1. Black tea

2. Cola

3. Coffee

4. Orange juice

5. Tomato juice

Miscellaneous:

1. Ketchup

2. Mayonnaise

3. Vinegar (except rice vinegar)

4. Pickles

5. Processed and canned foods

Chapter 5

28-day Meal Planning for Blood Type A

Week 1:

Day 1:

- Breakfast: Quinoa Porridge with Mixed Berries

- Snack: Sliced Apple with Almond Butter

- Lunch: Lentil and Vegetable Soup

- Snack: Greek Yogurt with a Drizzle of Honey (in moderation)

- Dinner: Baked Trout with Steamed Broccoli and Brown Rice

- Dessert: Chia Seed Pudding with Fresh Mango

Day 2:

- Breakfast: Green Smoothie with Kale, Banana, and Almond Milk

- Snack: Handful of Walnuts

- Lunch: Tofu Stir-Fry with Assorted Vegetables and Quinoa

- Snack: Carrot Sticks with Hummus

- Dinner: Chickpea and Spinach Curry with Brown Rice

- Dessert: Fresh Berry Parfait with Almond Milk Yogurt

Day 3:

- Breakfast: Oatmeal with Sliced Apples and Flaxseeds

- Snack: Rice Cake with Avocado Slices

- Lunch: Turkey and Vegetable Lettuce Wraps

- Snack: Mango Smoothie with Chia Seeds

- Dinner: Grilled Salmon with Quinoa and Steamed Asparagus

- Dessert: Dark Chocolate (in moderation)

Day 4:

- Breakfast: Greek Yogurt Smoothie with Berries

- Snack: Handful of Pumpkin Seeds

- Lunch: Spinach and Chickpea Salad with Lemon-Tahini Dressing

- Snack: Banana with Almond Butter

- Dinner: Stir-fried tempeh with Broccoli and Brown Rice

- Dessert: Baked Apples with Cinnamon

Day 5:

- Breakfast: Chia Seed Pudding with Coconut Milk and Pineapple

- Snack: Mixed Berry Bowl

- Lunch: Quinoa and Black Bean Bowl with Avocado

- Snack: Celery Sticks with Peanut Butter (in moderation)

- Dinner: Miso-glazed trout with Roasted Sweet Potatoes and Asparagus

- Dessert: Coconut Milk Rice Pudding

Day 6:

- Breakfast: Smoothie Bowl with Mixed Berries, Banana, and Almond Milk

- Snack: Apple Slices with Cinnamon

- Lunch: Lentil and Vegetable Curry with Brown Rice

- Snack: Cherry Tomatoes with Balsamic Glaze

- Dinner: Tofu and Vegetable Kebabs with Quinoa

- Dessert: Frozen Grapes

Day 7:

- Breakfast: Almond Butter Toast with Sliced Strawberries

- Snack: Handful of Almonds

- Lunch: Quinoa-stuffed bell Peppers with a Side of Mixed Greens

- Snack: Pear Slices with Goat Cheese (in moderation)

- Dinner: Baked Chicken with Lemon and Herbs, Quinoa, and Roasted Brussels Sprouts

- Dessert: Vanilla Almond Chia Pudding

Week 2:

Day 8:

- Breakfast: Buckwheat Pancakes with Fresh Blueberries

- Snack: Carrot and Cucumber Sticks with Hummus

- Lunch: Chickpea and Vegetable Stir-Fry with Brown Rice

- Snack: Mixed Berry Smoothie

- Dinner: Grilled Trout with Lemon-Dill Sauce, Quinoa, and Steamed Broccoli

- Dessert: Mango Sorbet

Day 9:

- Breakfast: Avocado and Tomato on Spelt Toast

- Snack: Rice Cake with Almond Butter

- Lunch: Spinach and Feta Omelet with a Side of Steamed Asparagus

- Snack: Fresh Fruit Salad

- Dinner: Stir-fried tempeh with Vegetables and Brown Rice

- Dessert: Raspberry Chia Jam with Rice Cakes

Day 10:

- Breakfast: Banana and Almond Smoothie with a Handful of Spinach

- Snack: Mixed Nuts Trail Mix

- Lunch: Turkey and Vegetable Stir-Fry with Quinoa

- Snack: Celery Sticks with Sunflower Seed Butter (in moderation)

- Dinner: Miso Soup with Seaweed, Tofu, and Brown Rice

- Dessert: Baked Pears with Cinnamon

Day 11:

- Breakfast: Overnight Oats with Sliced Peaches and a Dash of Cinnamon

- Snack: Orange Slices

- Lunch: Quinoa Salad with Mixed Greens and Lemon Vinaigrette

- Snack: Blueberry Smoothie

- Dinner: Grilled Chicken with Quinoa and Sautéed Swiss Chard

- Dessert: Dark Chocolate-Dipped Strawberries

Day 12:

- Breakfast: Fresh Fruit Salad with a Dollop of Greek Yogurt (in moderation)

- Snack: Handful of Pistachios

- Lunch: Lentil Salad with Tomatoes, Cucumbers, and Feta Cheese (in moderation)

- Snack: Apple and Almond Butter Sandwich

- Dinner: Baked Salmon with Quinoa and Roasted Sweet Potatoes

- Dessert: Coconut Chia Seed Pudding

Day 13:

- Breakfast: Quinoa and Almond Milk Parfait with Berries

- Snack: Pineapple Spears

- Lunch: Turkey and Avocado Wrap with a Side of Mixed Greens

- Snack: Frozen Banana Bites

- Dinner: Stir-fried tofu with Vegetables and Brown Rice

- Dessert: Vanilla Almond Date Balls

Day 14:

- Breakfast: Green Tea Smoothie with Mango and Spinach

- Snack: Watermelon Cubes

- Lunch: Chickpea and Spinach Salad with Tahini Dressing

- Snack: Cherry Tomatoes with Guacamole

- Dinner: Grilled Trout with Quinoa and Steamed Asparagus

- Dessert: Lemon Sorbet

Week 3:

Day 15:

- Breakfast: Buckwheat Waffles with Mixed Berries

- Snack: Handful of Cashews

- Lunch: Quinoa and Black Bean Bowl with Avocado

- Snack: Carrot Sticks with Hummus

- Dinner: Miso-glazed salmon with Roasted Sweet Potatoes and Broccoli

- Dessert: Raspberry Almond Thumbprint Cookies

Day 16:

- Breakfast: Acai Bowl with Granola and Sliced Kiwi

- Snack: Mango Slices

- Lunch: Spinach and Feta Stuffed Mushrooms with a Side Salad

- Snack: Rice Cake with Almond Butter and Banana Slices

- Dinner: Quinoa-Crusted Chicken Tenders with Roasted Vegetables

- Dessert: Mixed Berry Sorbet

Day 17:

- Breakfast: Avocado and Berry Smoothie

- Snack: Cucumber Slices with Hummus

- Lunch: Lentil and Vegetable Curry with Brown Rice

- Snack: Greek Yogurt with Mixed Berries (in moderation)

- Dinner: Tofu and Vegetable Kebabs with Quinoa

- Dessert: Dark Chocolate-Dipped Apricots

Day 18:

- Breakfast: Chia Seed Pudding Parfait with Fresh Mango

- Snack: Almond Butter and Banana Roll-Ups

- Lunch: Quinoa-stuffed bell Peppers with a Side Salad

- Snack: Handful of Strawberries

- Dinner: Baked Chicken with Lemon and Herbs, Quinoa, and Roasted Brussels Sprouts

- Dessert: Coconut Milk Rice Pudding

Day 19:

- Breakfast: Pineapple and Coconut Smoothie Bowl

- Snack: Watermelon Cubes

- Lunch: Chickpea and Vegetable Stir-Fry with Brown Rice

- Snack: Pear Slices with Goat Cheese (in moderation)

- Dinner: Grilled Trout with Lemon-Dill Sauce, Quinoa, and Steamed Broccoli

- Dessert: Mango Sorbet

Day 20:

- Breakfast: Almond Butter Toast with Sliced Strawberries

- Snack: Handful of Walnuts

- Lunch: Spinach and Chickpea Salad with Lemon-Tahini Dressing

- Snack: Banana and Almond Smoothie

- Dinner: Stir-fried tempeh with Vegetables and Brown Rice

- Dessert: Dark Chocolate (in moderation)

Week 4 :

Day 21:

- Breakfast: Greek Yogurt Smoothie with Berries

- Snack: Handful of Almonds

- Lunch: Quinoa and Black Bean Bowl with Avocado

- Snack: Celery Sticks with Hummus

- Dinner: Grilled Salmon with Quinoa and Steamed Broccoli

- Dessert: Mango Sorbet

Day 22:

- Breakfast: Buckwheat Pancakes with Fresh Blueberries

- Snack: Rice Cake with Almond Butter

- Lunch: Chickpea and Vegetable Stir-Fry with Brown Rice

- Snack: Fresh Fruit Salad

- Dinner: Miso Soup with Seaweed, Tofu, and Brown Rice

- Dessert: Dark Chocolate (in moderation)

Day 23:

- Breakfast: Avocado and Tomato on Spelt Toast

- Snack: Mixed Nuts Trail Mix

- Lunch: Spinach and Feta Omelet with a Side of Steamed Asparagus

- Snack: Mango Smoothie with Chia Seeds

- Dinner: Baked Trout with Lemon-Dill Sauce, Quinoa, and Roasted Brussels Sprouts

- Dessert: Coconut Chia Seed Pudding

Day 24:

- Breakfast: Banana and Almond Smoothie with a Handful of Spinach

- Snack: Handful of Pistachios

- Lunch: Quinoa-stuffed bell Peppers with a Side of Mixed Greens

- Snack: Cherry Tomatoes with Guacamole

- Dinner: Grilled Chicken with Quinoa and Sautéed Swiss Chard

- Dessert: Raspberry Almond Thumbprint Cookies

Day 25:

- Breakfast: Acai Bowl with Granola and Sliced Kiwi

- Snack: Apple Slices with Cinnamon

- Lunch: Lentil and Vegetable Curry with Brown Rice

- Snack: Pear Slices with Goat Cheese (in moderation)

- Dinner: Tofu and Vegetable Kebabs with Quinoa

- Dessert: Vanilla Almond Date Balls

Day 26:

- Breakfast: Fresh Fruit Salad with a Dollop of Greek Yogurt (in moderation)

- Snack: Rice Cake with Avocado Slices

- Lunch: Turkey and Avocado Wrap with a Side of Mixed Greens

- Snack: Frozen Banana Bites

- Dinner: Stir-fried tempeh with Vegetables and Brown Rice

- Dessert: Raspberry Chia Jam with Rice Cakes

Day 27:

- Breakfast: Green Tea Smoothie with Mango and Spinach

- Snack: Orange Slices

- Lunch: Chickpea and Spinach Salad with Tahini Dressing

- Snack: Blueberry Smoothie

- Dinner: Grilled Trout with Quinoa and Steamed Asparagus

- Dessert: Dark Chocolate-Dipped Strawberries

Day 28:

- Breakfast: Quinoa Porridge with Mixed Berries

- Snack: Sliced Apple with Almond Butter

- Lunch: Lentil and Vegetable Soup

- Snack: Greek Yogurt with a Drizzle of Honey (in moderation)

- Dinner: Baked Trout with Steamed Broccoli and Brown Rice

- Dessert: Chia Seed Pudding with Fresh Mango

Chapter 6

Blood Type A-Breakfast Friendly Recipes

Quinoa Porridge with Mixed Berries

Ingredients:

- 1/2 cup quinoa

- 1 cup almond milk

- Mixed berries (strawberries, blueberries, raspberries)

- 1 tablespoon honey (optional)

Instructions:

1. Rinse quinoa and cook it in almond milk until soft.

2. Top with mixed berries and drizzle honey if desired.

Nutritional Information (per serving):

- Calories: 300

- Protein: 10g

- Fat: 6g

- Carbohydrates: 50g

- Fiber: 7g

Green Smoothie with Kale and Banana

Ingredients:

- 1 cup kale

- 1 banana

- 1/2 cup almond milk

- Ice cubes

Instructions:

1. Blend kale, banana, and almond milk until smooth.

2. Add ice cubes and blend again.

Nutritional Information (per serving):

- Calories: 150

- Protein: 4g

- Fat: 2g

- Carbohydrates: 30g

- Fiber: 5g

Oatmeal with Sliced Apples and Flaxseeds

Ingredients:

- 1/2 cup oats

- 1 cup almond milk

- 1 apple, sliced

- 1 tablespoon flaxseeds

Instructions:

1. Cook oats in almond milk.

2. Top with sliced apples and sprinkle with flaxseeds.

Nutritional Information (per serving):

- Calories: 250

- Protein: 5g

- Fat: 4g

- Carbohydrates: 45g

- Fiber: 8g

Greek Yogurt Smoothie with Berries

Ingredients:

- 1/2 cup Greek yogurt

- 1/2 cup mixed berries

- 1/2 cup almond milk

- 1 tablespoon chia seeds

Instructions:

1. Blend Greek yogurt, mixed berries, and almond milk.

2. Stir in chia seeds.

Nutritional Information (per serving):

- Calories: 200

- Protein: 15g

- Fat: 7g

- Carbohydrates: 20g

- Fiber: 6g

Chia Seed Pudding with Coconut Milk and Pineapple

Ingredients:

- 2 tablespoons chia seeds

- 1/2 cup coconut milk

- 1/2 cup diced pineapple

- Shredded coconut (for topping)

Instructions:

1. Mix chia seeds with coconut milk and refrigerate overnight.

2. Top with diced pineapple and shredded coconut.

Nutritional Information (per serving):

- Calories: 220

- Protein: 5g

- Fat: 15g

- Carbohydrates: 20g

- Fiber: 8g

Buckwheat Pancakes with Fresh Blueberries

Ingredients:

- 1/2 cup buckwheat flour

- 1/2 cup almond milk

- 1 egg

- Fresh blueberries (for topping)

Instructions:

1. Mix buckwheat flour, almond milk, and egg to make batter.

2. Cook pancakes and top with fresh blueberries.

Nutritional Information (per serving):

- Calories: 220

- Protein: 8g

- Fat: 6g

- Carbohydrates: 30g

- Fiber: 5g

Smoothie Bowl with Mixed Berries and Banana

Ingredients:

- 1 frozen banana

- 1/2 cup mixed berries

- 1/2 cup almond milk

- Granola and sliced kiwi (for topping)

Instructions:

1. Blend frozen banana, mixed berries, and almond milk until smooth.

2. Pour into a bowl and top with granola and sliced kiwi.

Nutritional Information (per serving):

- Calories: 280

- Protein: 6g

- Fat: 4g

- Carbohydrates: 50g

- Fiber: 9g

Avocado and Tomato on Spelt Toast

Ingredients:

- 1 slice spelt bread

- 1/2 avocado, sliced

- 1 tomato, sliced

- Sprinkle of sea salt

Instructions:

1. Toast spelt bread.

2. Top with sliced avocado and tomato. Sprinkle with sea salt.

Nutritional Information (per serving):

- Calories: 200

- Protein: 5g

- Fat: 10g

- Carbohydrates: 25g

- Fiber: 7g

Chia Seed Pudding Parfait with Fresh Mango

Ingredients:

- 2 tablespoons chia seeds

- 1/2 cup almond milk

- 1/2 cup diced mango

- Granola (for layering)

Instructions:

1. Mix chia seeds with almond milk and refrigerate until set.

2. In a glass, layer chia pudding with diced mango and granola.

Nutritional Information (per serving):

- Calories: 240

- Protein: 6g

- Fat: 10g

- Carbohydrates: 30g

- Fiber: 8g

Green Tea Smoothie with Mango and Spinach

Ingredients:

- 1 cup brewed green tea (cooled)

- 1/2 cup mango chunks

- Handful of spinach

- 1/2 banana

Instructions:

1. Blend green tea, mango chunks, spinach, and banana until smooth.

2. Pour into a glass and enjoy.

Nutritional Information (per serving):

- Calories: 180

- Protein: 3g

- Fat: 1g

- Carbohydrates: 40g

- Fiber: 6g

Pineapple and Coconut Smoothie Bowl

Ingredients:

- 1/2 cup pineapple chunks

- 1/2 cup coconut milk

- 1/4 cup rolled oats

- Shredded coconut and sliced banana (for topping)

Instructions:

1. Blend pineapple chunks, coconut milk, and rolled oats until smooth.

2. Pour into a bowl and top with shredded coconut and sliced banana.

Nutritional Information (per serving):

- Calories: 250

- Protein: 4g

- Fat: 10g

- Carbohydrates: 35g

- Fiber: 7g

Acai Bowl with Granola and Sliced Kiwi

Ingredients:

- 1 packet frozen acai

- 1/2 cup almond milk

- Granola and sliced kiwi (for topping)

- Chia seeds (optional)

Instructions:

1. Blend frozen acai with almond milk until smooth.

2. Pour into a bowl and top with granola, sliced kiwi, and chia seeds if desired.

Nutritional Information (per serving):

- Calories: 300

- Protein: 5g

- Fat: 12g

- Carbohydrates: 40g

- Fiber: 8g

Almond Butter Toast with Sliced Strawberries

Ingredients:

- 1 slice whole grain bread

- 2 tablespoons almond butter

- Fresh strawberries, sliced

Instructions:

1. Toast whole grain bread.

2. Spread almond butter on the toast and top with sliced strawberries.

Nutritional Information (per serving):

- Calories: 280

- Protein: 7g

- Fat: 15g

- Carbohydrates: 30g

- Fiber: 7g

Chapter 7

Blood Type A-Lunch Friendly Recipes

Lentil and Vegetable Soup

Ingredients:

- 1 cup lentils

- 2 carrots, diced

- 2 celery stalks, chopped

- 1 onion, diced

- 4 cups vegetable broth

- 2 cloves garlic, minced

- 1 teaspoon cumin

- Salt and pepper to taste

Instructions:

1. In a pot, sauté onion, carrots, and celery until softened.

2. Add garlic, lentils, cumin, and vegetable broth.

3. Simmer until lentils are cooked. Season with salt and pepper.

Nutritional Information (per serving):

- Calories: 250

- Protein: 15g

- Fat: 2g

- Carbohydrates: 45g

- Fiber: 12g

Turkey and Vegetable Lettuce Wraps

Ingredients:

- 1 lb ground turkey

- 1 bell pepper, diced

- 1 zucchini, grated

- 1 cup mushrooms, chopped

- Lettuce leaves for wrapping

- 2 tablespoons soy sauce

- 1 teaspoon ginger, grated

Instructions:

1. Brown ground turkey in a pan.

2. Add bell pepper, zucchini, and mushrooms. Cook until vegetables are tender.

3. Stir in soy sauce and ginger. Serve in lettuce wraps.

Nutritional Information (per serving):

- Calories: 280

- Protein: 25g

- Fat: 12g

- Carbohydrates: 18g

- Fiber: 5g

Chickpea and Spinach Salad with Lemon-Tahini Dressing

Ingredients:

- 1 can chickpeas, drained and rinsed

- 2 cups spinach

- 1 cucumber, diced

- 1 cup cherry tomatoes, halved

- 1/4 cup red onion, thinly sliced

Lemon-Tahini Dressing:

- 2 tablespoons tahini

- Juice of 1 lemon

- 1 tablespoon olive oil

- Salt and pepper to taste

Instructions:

1. In a bowl, combine chickpeas, spinach, cucumber, tomatoes, and red onion.

2. Whisk together dressing ingredients and pour over the salad.

Nutritional Information (per serving):

- Calories: 320

- Protein: 12g

- Fat: 18g

- Carbohydrates: 35g

- Fiber: 9g

Tofu Stir-Fry with Assorted Vegetables and Quinoa

Ingredients:

- 1 cup quinoa, cooked

- 1 block tofu, cubed

- 2 cups broccoli florets

- 1 bell pepper, sliced

- 1 carrot, julienned

- 2 tablespoons soy sauce

- 1 tablespoon sesame oil

Instructions:

1. Sauté tofu in sesame oil until golden.

2. Add broccoli, bell pepper, and carrot. Cook until vegetables are tender.

3. Stir in soy sauce and serve over cooked quinoa.

Nutritional Information (per serving):

- Calories: 350

- Protein: 18g

- Fat: 15g

- Carbohydrates: 40g

- Fiber: 7g

Quinoa and Black Bean Bowl with Avocado

Ingredients:

- 1 cup quinoa, cooked

- 1 can black beans, drained and rinsed

- 1 avocado, diced

- 1 cup corn kernels

- 1/4 cup cilantro, chopped

- Juice of 2 limes

Instructions:

1. Mix cooked quinoa, black beans, avocado, corn, cilantro, and lime juice.

2. Toss until well combined.

Nutritional Information (per serving):

- Calories: 320

- Protein: 12g

- Fat: 12g

- Carbohydrates: 45g

- Fiber: 12g

Spinach and Chickpea Salad with Lemon-Tahini Dressing

Ingredients:

- 2 cups spinach

- 1 can chickpeas, drained and rinsed

- 1 cucumber, diced

- 1 cup cherry tomatoes, halved

- 1/4 cup red onion, thinly sliced

Lemon-Tahini Dressing:

- 2 tablespoons tahini

- Juice of 1 lemon

- 1 tablespoon olive oil

- Salt and pepper to taste

Instructions:

1. Combine spinach, chickpeas, cucumber, tomatoes, and red onion in a bowl.

2. Whisk together dressing ingredients and toss with the salad.

Nutritional Information (per serving):

- Calories: 290

- Protein: 11g

- Fat: 16g

- Carbohydrates: 32g

- Fiber: 8g

Miso-glazed salmon with Roasted Sweet Potatoes and Asparagus

Ingredients:

- 2 salmon fillets

- 2 tablespoons miso paste

- 1 tablespoon maple syrup

- 2 sweet potatoes, cubed

- 1 bunch asparagus, trimmed

- 2 tablespoons olive oil

Instructions:

1. Mix miso paste and maple syrup. Coat salmon with the mixture.

2. Toss sweet potatoes and asparagus in olive oil. Roast until tender.

Nutritional Information (per serving):

- Calories: 400

- Protein: 25g

- Fat: 20g

- Carbohydrates: 30g

- Fiber: 7g

Chickpea and Vegetable Stir-Fry with Brown Rice

Ingredients:

- 1 cup brown rice, cooked

- 1 can chickpeas, drained and rinsed

- 1 cup broccoli florets

- 1 bell pepper, sliced

- 1 carrot, julienned

- 2 tablespoons soy sauce

- 1 tablespoon sesame oil

Instructions:

1. Sauté chickpeas, broccoli, bell pepper, and carrot in sesame oil.

2. Stir in soy sauce and serve over cooked brown rice.

Nutritional Information (per serving):

- Calories: 340

- Protein: 15g

- Fat: 12g

- Carbohydrates: 45g

- Fiber: 9g

Turkey and Avocado Wrap with a Side of Mixed Greens

Ingredients:

- 1 whole grain wrap

- 1/2 lb sliced turkey breast

- 1 avocado, sliced

- Mixed greens

- Hummus (optional)

Instructions:

1. Lay out the wrap and layer with turkey, avocado, mixed greens, and hummus if desired.

2. Roll up the wrap and slice it in half.

Nutritional Information (per serving):

- Calories: 380

- Protein: 25g

- Fat: 15g

- Carbohydrates: 35g

- Fiber: 8g

Quinoa-Stuffed Bell Peppers with a Side of Mixed Greens

Ingredients:

- 2 bell peppers, halved

- 1 cup quinoa, cooked

- 1 can black beans, drained and rinsed

- 1 cup corn kernels

- 1/2 cup salsa

Instructions:

1. Mix cooked quinoa, black beans, corn, and salsa.

2. Stuff bell peppers with the quinoa mixture. Bake until the peppers are tender.

Nutritional Information (per serving):

- Calories: 320

- Protein: 12g

- Fat: 8g

- Carbohydrates: 50g

- Fiber: 12g

Chickpea and Vegetable Curry with Brown Rice

Ingredients:

- 1 cup brown rice, cooked

- 1 can chickpeas, drained and rinsed

- 1 cup cauliflower florets

- 1 cup green peas

- 1 onion, diced

- 2 tomatoes, chopped

- 1 tablespoon curry powder

Instructions:

1. Sauté onion, chickpeas, cauliflower, and green peas in a pan.

2. Add tomatoes and curry powder. Simmer until vegetables are tender. Serve over brown rice.

Nutritional Information (per serving):

- Calories: 380

- Protein: 15g

- Fat: 8g

- Carbohydrates: 65g

- Fiber: 10g

Chapter 8

Blood Type A-Dinner Friendly Recipes

Stir-fried tempeh with Vegetables and Brown Rice

Ingredients:

- 1 cup brown rice, cooked

- 1 pack tempeh, cubed

- 2 cups mixed vegetables (broccoli, bell peppers, snap peas)

- 2 tablespoons soy sauce

- 1 tablespoon sesame oil

Instructions:

1. Stir-fry tempeh and mixed vegetables in sesame oil.

2. Add soy sauce and cook until vegetables are tender. Serve over brown rice.

Nutritional Information (per serving):

- Calories: 360

- Protein: 18g

- Fat: 15g

- Carbohydrates: 45g

- Fiber: 9g

Grilled Salmon with Quinoa and Steamed Broccoli

Ingredients:

- 2 salmon fillets

- 1 cup quinoa, cooked

- 2 cups broccoli florets

- Lemon wedges for garnish

- Olive oil for brushing

Instructions:

1. Brush salmon with olive oil and grill until cooked.

2. Serve over quinoa with steamed broccoli. Garnish with lemon.

Nutritional Information (per serving):

- Calories: 420

- Protein: 30g

- Fat: 18g

- Carbohydrates: 35g

- Fiber: 7g

Grilled Trout with Lemon-Dill Sauce, Quinoa, and Steamed Asparagus

Ingredients:

- 2 trout fillets

- 1 lemon, juiced

- 2 tablespoons fresh dill, chopped

- 1 cup quinoa, cooked

- 1 bunch asparagus, steamed

Instructions:

1. Grill trout fillets and squeeze lemon juice over them.

2. Mix chopped dill with lemon juice. Serve trout over quinoa with steamed asparagus.

Nutritional Information (per serving):

- Calories: 400

- Protein: 30g

- Fat: 15g

- Carbohydrates: 35g

- Fiber: 8g

Baked Chicken with Rosemary, Sweet Potato Mash, and Green Beans

Ingredients:

- 2 chicken breasts

- 2 tablespoons olive oil

- 1 tablespoon fresh rosemary, chopped

- 2 sweet potatoes, mashed

- 2 cups green beans, steamed

Instructions:

1. Coat chicken with olive oil and sprinkle with chopped rosemary. Bake until cooked.

2. Serve over sweet potato mash with steamed green beans.

Nutritional Information (per serving):

- Calories: 380

- Protein: 25g

- Fat: 15g

- Carbohydrates: 30g

- Fiber: 8g

Quinoa-Stuffed Bell Peppers with Tomato Sauce

Ingredients:

- 4 bell peppers, halved

- 1 cup quinoa, cooked

- 1 can black beans, drained and rinsed

- 1 cup corn kernels

- 1 cup tomato sauce

Instructions:

1. Mix cooked quinoa, black beans, and corn. Stuff bell peppers.

2. Pour tomato sauce over the stuffed peppers and bake until the peppers are tender.

Nutritional Information (per serving):

- Calories: 320

- Protein: 12g

- Fat: 8g

- Carbohydrates: 50g

- Fiber: 12g

Chia Seed-Crusted Tofu with Sweet Potato Fries

Ingredients:

- 1 block tofu, sliced

- 2 tablespoons chia seeds

- 1 tablespoon olive oil

- 2 sweet potatoes, cut into fries

Instructions:

1. Coat tofu slices in chia seeds and bake until crispy.

2. Toss sweet potato fries in olive oil and bake until golden.

Nutritional Information (per serving):

- Calories: 380

- Protein: 18g

- Fat: 15g

- Carbohydrates: 50g

- Fiber: 12g

Lemon Garlic Shrimp with Quinoa and Roasted Brussels Sprouts

Ingredients:

- 1 lb shrimp, peeled and deveined

- 2 tablespoons olive oil

- 3 cloves garlic, minced

- 1 lemon, juiced

- 1 cup quinoa, cooked

- 2 cups Brussels sprouts, halved and roasted

Instructions:

1. Sauté shrimp in olive oil with minced garlic until cooked.

2. Drizzle lemon juice over the shrimp. Serve over quinoa with roasted Brussels sprouts.

Nutritional Information (per serving):

- Calories: 350

- Protein: 25g

- Fat: 15g

- Carbohydrates: 30g

- Fiber: 8g

Greek Salad with Grilled Chicken

Ingredients:

- 1 lb chicken breast, grilled and sliced

- 2 cups mixed greens

- 1 cucumber, diced

- 1 cup cherry tomatoes, halved

- 1/2 red onion, thinly sliced

- 1/2 cup feta cheese, crumbled

- Kalamata olives

- Greek dressing

Instructions:

1. Assemble mixed greens, cucumber, tomatoes, red onion, feta, and olives.

2. Top with grilled chicken and drizzle with Greek dressing.

Nutritional Information (per serving):

- Calories: 380

- Protein: 30g

- Fat: 15g

- Carbohydrates: 30g

- Fiber: 8g

Spaghetti Squash with Tomato Basil Sauce and Turkey Meatballs

Ingredients:

- 1 spaghetti squash, roasted and shredded

- 1 lb ground turkey

- 2 cups tomato basil sauce

- Fresh basil for garnish

- Parmesan cheese (optional)

Instructions:

1. Mix ground turkey and form into meatballs. Bake until cooked.

2. Serve turkey meatballs over spaghetti squash with tomato basil sauce. Garnish with fresh basil and Parmesan if desired.

Nutritional Information (per serving):

- Calories: 360

- Protein: 25g

- Fat: 12g

- Carbohydrates: 35g

- Fiber: 8g

Eggplant and Chickpea Stew with Brown Rice

Ingredients:

- 1 cup brown rice, cooked

- 1 eggplant, diced

- 1 can chickpeas, drained and rinsed

- 1 onion, diced

- 2 tomatoes, chopped

- 2 cloves garlic, minced

- 1 tablespoon cumin

- 1 teaspoon paprika

Instructions:

1. Sauté onion, eggplant, and garlic until softened.

2. Add chickpeas, tomatoes, cumin, and paprika. Simmer until

vegetables are tender. Serve over brown rice.

Nutritional Information (per serving):

- Calories: 340

- Protein: 12g

- Fat: 8g

- Carbohydrates: 60g

- Fiber: 10g

Mushroom and Spinach Stuffed Chicken Breast with Quinoa

Ingredients:

- 2 chicken breasts

- 1 cup quinoa, cooked

- 1 cup mushrooms, chopped

- 2 cups spinach, chopped

- 2 cloves garlic, minced

- 1 tablespoon olive oil

Instructions:

1. Sauté mushrooms, spinach, and garlic in olive oil until wilted.

2. Cut a pocket in each chicken breast and stuff with the mushroom and spinach mixture. Bake until cooked.

3. Serve over quinoa.

Nutritional Information (per serving):

- Calories: 380

- Protein: 30g

- Fat: 15g

- Carbohydrates: 35g

- Fiber: 8g

Salmon and Quinoa Salad with Lemon-Dill Dressing

Ingredients:

- 2 salmon fillets, grilled

- 1 cup quinoa, cooked

- 2 cups mixed greens

- 1 cucumber, sliced

- 1/4 cup red onion, thinly sliced

Lemon-Dill Dressing:

- 2 tablespoons olive oil

- Juice of 1 lemon

- 1 tablespoon fresh dill, chopped

- Salt and pepper to taste

Instructions:

1. Mix quinoa, mixed greens, cucumber, and red onion in a bowl.

2. Top with grilled salmon. Whisk together dressing ingredients and drizzle over the salad.

Nutritional Information (per serving):

- Calories: 400

- Protein: 30g

- Fat: 18g

- Carbohydrates: 30g

- Fiber: 8g

Sweet Potato and Black Bean Chili

Ingredients:

- 2 sweet potatoes, diced

- 1 can black beans, drained and rinsed

- 1 can diced tomatoes

- 1 onion, diced

- 2 cloves garlic, minced

- 1 tablespoon chili powder

- 1 teaspoon cumin

Instructions:

1. Sauté onion and garlic until softened.

2. Add sweet potatoes, black beans, diced tomatoes, chili powder, and cumin. Simmer until sweet potatoes are tender.

Nutritional Information (per serving):

- Calories: 350

- Protein: 12g

- Fat: 8g

- Carbohydrates: 60g

- Fiber: 12g

Chapter 9

Blood Type A-Snacks Friendly Recipes

Hummus and Veggie Sticks

Ingredients:

- 1 cup hummus

- Carrot sticks

- Cucumber slices

- Bell pepper strips

Instructions:

1. Arrange veggie sticks on a plate.

2. Serve with hummus for dipping.

Nutritional Information (per serving):

- Calories: 150

- Protein: 5g

- Fat: 10g

- Carbohydrates: 15g

- Fiber: 6g

Greek Yogurt Parfait with Berries

Ingredients:

- 1 cup Greek yogurt

- Mixed berries (blueberries, strawberries, raspberries)

- Granola

Instructions:

1. Layer Greek yogurt, berries, and granola in a glass.

2. Repeat layers. Enjoy!

Nutritional Information (per serving):

- Calories: 250

- Protein: 18g

- Fat: 8g

- Carbohydrates: 30g

- Fiber: 5g

Avocado and Tomato Salsa with Rice Cakes

Ingredients:

- 1 ripe avocado, mashed

- 1 cup cherry tomatoes, diced

- 1/4 red onion, finely chopped

- Rice cakes

Instructions:

1. Mix mashed avocado, tomatoes, and red onion.

2. Spread the mixture on rice cakes.

Nutritional Information (per serving):

- Calories: 180

- Protein: 3g

- Fat: 10g

- Carbohydrates: 20g

- Fiber: 5g

Mixed Nuts and Dried Fruits

Ingredients:

- 1/2 cup mixed nuts (almonds, walnuts, cashews)
- 1/4 cup dried fruits (apricots, figs, dates)

Instructions:

1. Combine mixed nuts and dried fruits in a bowl.
2. Portion into snack-sized servings.

Nutritional Information (per serving):

- Calories: 200
- Protein: 5g
- Fat: 15g
- Carbohydrates: 15g
- Fiber: 3g

Cottage Cheese and Pineapple Cups

Ingredients:

- 1 cup cottage cheese

- Fresh pineapple chunks

Instructions:

1. Fill small cups with cottage cheese.

2. Top with fresh pineapple chunks.

Nutritional Information (per serving):

- Calories: 180

- Protein: 15g

- Fat: 8g

- Carbohydrates: 15g

- Fiber: 1g

Rice Cake with Almond Butter and Banana Slices

Ingredients:

- Rice cakes

- Almond butter

- Banana, sliced

Instructions:

1. Spread almond butter on rice cakes.

2. Top with banana slices.

Nutritional Information (per serving):

- Calories: 200

- Protein: 4g

- Fat: 10g

- Carbohydrates: 25g

- Fiber: 3g

Edamame with Sea Salt

Ingredients:

- 1 cup edamame, steamed

- Sea salt to taste

Instructions:

1. Steam edamame until tender.

2. Sprinkle with sea salt.

Nutritional Information (per serving):

- Calories: 150

- Protein: 12g

- Fat: 8g

- Carbohydrates: 10g

- Fiber: 6g

Kale Chips with Nutritional Yeast

Ingredients:

- 1 bunch of kale, stems removed

- 1 tablespoon olive oil

- 2 tablespoons nutritional yeast

Instructions:

1. Toss kale in olive oil and sprinkle with nutritional yeast.

2. Bake until crispy.

Nutritional Information (per serving):

- Calories: 120

- Protein: 5g

- Fat: 8g

- Carbohydrates: 10g

- Fiber: 3g

Chia Seed Pudding with Berries

Ingredients:

- 2 tablespoons chia seeds
- 1 cup almond milk
- Mixed berries for topping

Instructions:

1. Mix chia seeds and almond milk. Let it sit until it thickens.
2. Top with mixed berries.

Nutritional Information (per serving):

- Calories: 150
- Protein: 5g
- Fat: 10g
- Carbohydrates: 15g
- Fiber: 8g

Apple Slices with Almond Butter and Cinnamon

Ingredients:

- Apple, sliced

- Almond butter

- Ground cinnamon

Instructions:

1. Spread almond butter on apple slices.

2. Sprinkle with ground cinnamon.

Nutritional Information (per serving):

- Calories: 180

- Protein: 3g

- Fat: 10g

- Carbohydrates: 20g

- Fiber: 5g

Roasted Red Pepper Hummus with Pita Chips

Ingredients:

- 1 cup roasted red pepper hummus

- Whole grain pita chips

Instructions:

1. Serve roasted red pepper hummus with whole-grain pita chips.

Nutritional Information (per serving):

- Calories: 200
- Protein: 5g
- Fat: 10g
- Carbohydrates: 25g
- Fiber: 6g

Cucumber and Tzatziki Bites

Ingredients:

- Cucumber, sliced
- Tzatziki sauce

Instructions:

1. Top cucumber slices with a dollop of tzatziki sauce.

Nutritional Information (per serving):

- Calories: 80
- Protein: 3g

- Fat: 5g

- Carbohydrates: 8g

- Fiber: 1g

Chocolate Covered Strawberries

Ingredients:

- Strawberries

- Dark chocolate melted

Instructions:

1. Dip strawberries in melted dark chocolate.

2. Place on parchment paper and let it cool.

Nutritional Information (per serving):

- Calories: 150

- Protein: 2g

- Fat: 8g

- Carbohydrates: 20g

- Fiber: 4g

Turmeric Roasted Chickpeas

Ingredients:

- 1 can chickpeas, drained and rinsed
- 1 tablespoon olive oil
- 1 teaspoon turmeric
- Sea salt to taste

Instructions:

1. Toss chickpeas in olive oil, turmeric, and sea salt.
2. Roast until crispy.

Nutritional Information (per serving):

- Calories: 180
- Protein: 7g
- Fat: 8g
- Carbohydrates: 20g
- Fiber: 5g

Chapter 10

Blood Type A-Dessert Friendly Recipes

Mixed Berry and Almond Parfait

Ingredients:

- 1 cup mixed berries (blueberries, strawberries, raspberries)
- 1/2 cup almond slices
- 1 cup Greek yogurt
- Honey for drizzling

Instructions:

1. In a glass, layer Greek yogurt, mixed berries, and almond slices.
2. Drizzle with honey. Repeat layers.

Nutritional Information (per serving):

- Calories: 250
- Protein: 15g
- Fat: 12g
- Carbohydrates: 25g
- Fiber: 5g

Chia Seed Pudding with Mango

Ingredients:

- 2 tablespoons chia seeds
- 1 cup almond milk
- 1 ripe mango, diced

Instructions:

1. Mix chia seeds and almond milk. Let it sit until it thickens.
2. Top with diced mango.

Nutritional Information (per serving):

- Calories: 180
- Protein: 5g
- Fat: 10g
- Carbohydrates: 20g
- Fiber: 8g

Coconut and Pineapple Sorbet

Ingredients:

- 2 cups frozen pineapple chunks
- 1 can coconut milk

- 1 tablespoon agave syrup

Instructions:

1. Blend frozen pineapple, coconut milk, and agave syrup until smooth.
2. Freeze until firm.

Nutritional Information (per serving):

- Calories: 200
- Protein: 2g
- Fat: 15g
- Carbohydrates: 20g
- Fiber: 2g

Avocado Chocolate Mousse

Ingredients:

- 2 ripe avocados
- 1/4 cup cocoa powder
- 1/4 cup maple syrup
- 1 teaspoon vanilla extract

Instructions:

1. Blend avocados, cocoa powder, maple syrup, and vanilla extract until smooth.
2. Chill before serving.

Nutritional Information (per serving):

- Calories: 220
- Protein: 3g
- Fat: 15g
- Carbohydrates: 25g
- Fiber: 7g

Baked Apples with Cinnamon and Walnuts

Ingredients:

- 2 apples, cored and halved
- 1 tablespoon melted coconut oil
- 1 teaspoon cinnamon
- 1/4 cup chopped walnuts

Instructions:

1. Preheat oven to 350°F (175°C).

2. Brush apple halves with melted coconut oil, sprinkle with cinnamon, and top with chopped walnuts.

3. Bake until the apples are tender.

Nutritional Information (per serving):

- Calories: 180
- Protein: 2g
- Fat: 10g
- Carbohydrates: 25g
- Fiber: 5g

Mint Chocolate Avocado Popsicles

Ingredients:

- 2 ripe avocados
- 1/4 cup cocoa powder
- 1/4 cup maple syrup
- Fresh mint leaves

Instructions:

1. Blend avocados, cocoa powder, and maple syrup until smooth.

2. Stir in chopped mint leaves.

3. Pour into popsicle molds and freeze.

Nutritional Information (per serving):

- Calories: 180

- Protein: 3g

- Fat: 15g

- Carbohydrates: 25g

- Fiber: 7g

Banana-Oat Cookies

Ingredients:

- 2 ripe bananas, mashed

- 1 cup rolled oats

- 1/4 cup almond butter

- 1/4 cup raisins

Instructions:

1. Preheat oven to 350°F (175°C).

2. Mix mashed bananas, rolled oats, almond butter, and raisins.

3. Drop spoonfuls onto a baking sheet and bake until golden.

Nutritional Information (per serving):

- Calories: 160
- Protein: 4g
- Fat: 8g
- Carbohydrates: 20g
- Fiber: 4g

Strawberry Coconut Chia Popsicles

Ingredients:

- 1 cup strawberries, pureed
- 1 can of coconut milk
- 2 tablespoons chia seeds

Instructions:

1. Mix strawberry puree, coconut milk, and chia seeds.
2. Pour into popsicle molds and freeze.

Nutritional Information (per serving):

- Calories: 180

- Protein: 3g

- Fat: 15g

- Carbohydrates: 20g

- Fiber: 6g

Peach and Almond Crisp

Ingredients:

- 4 ripe peaches, sliced

- 1 cup almond flour

- 1/4 cup coconut oil

- 1/4 cup maple syrup

- 1 teaspoon cinnamon

Instructions:

1. Preheat oven to 350°F (175°C).

2. Arrange peach slices in a baking dish.

3. In a bowl, mix almond flour, melted coconut oil, maple syrup, and cinnamon.

4. Sprinkle the mixture over the peaches and bake until golden.

Nutritional Information (per serving):

- Calories: 220
- Protein: 4g
- Fat: 15g
- Carbohydrates: 25g
- Fiber: 5g

Raspberry Coconut Chia Pudding

Ingredients:

- 1/4 cup chia seeds
- 1 cup coconut milk
- 1/2 cup raspberries
- 1 tablespoon honey

Instructions:

1. Mix chia seeds and coconut milk. Let it sit until it thickens.
2. Layer with raspberries and drizzle honey.

Nutritional Information (per serving):

- Calories: 200

- Protein: 3g
- Fat: 15g
- Carbohydrates: 20g
- Fiber: 8g

Almond Butter and Banana Ice Cream

Ingredients:

- 3 ripe bananas, frozen
- 1/4 cup almond butter
- 1 teaspoon vanilla extract

Instructions:

1. Blend frozen bananas, almond butter, and vanilla extract until creamy.
2. Freeze for a firmer texture.

Nutritional Information (per serving):

- Calories: 220
- Protein: 4g
- Fat: 15g
- Carbohydrates: 25g

- Fiber: 4g

Blueberry and Oat Muffins

Ingredients:

- 1 cup rolled oats
- 1 cup almond flour
- 1/4 cup coconut oil
- 1/4 cup maple syrup
- 1 cup blueberries

Instructions:

1. Preheat oven to 350°F (175°C).
2. Mix rolled oats, almond flour, melted coconut oil, maple syrup, and blueberries.
3. Spoon into muffin cups and bake until golden.

Nutritional Information (per serving):

- Calories: 230
- Protein: 5g
- Fat: 15g

- Carbohydrates: 25g
- Fiber: 5g

Coconut and Lime Energy Bites

Ingredients:

- 1 cup shredded coconut
- 1/2 cup cashews
- Zest and juice of 2 limes
- 1/4 cup dates, pitted

Instructions:

1. Blend shredded coconut, cashews, lime zest, lime juice, and dates until a sticky mixture forms.
2. Roll into bite-sized balls and refrigerate.

Nutritional Information (per serving):

- Calories: 180
- Protein: 3g
- Fat: 15g
- Carbohydrates: 15g

- Fiber: 4g

Chocolate-Covered Almond Clusters

Ingredients:

- 1 cup almonds
- 1/2 cup dark chocolate, melted

Instructions:

1. Mix almonds with melted dark chocolate.
2. Drop spoonfuls onto parchment paper and let it cool.

Nutritional Information (per serving):

- Calories: 200
- Protein: 5g
- Fat: 15g
- Carbohydrates: 15g
- Fiber: 3g

Chapter 11

Conclusion

In conclusion, the Blood Type A Cookbook and Food List Guide provides a comprehensive and tailored approach to nutrition, recognizing the unique dietary needs and preferences associated with Blood Type A individuals. Rooted in the belief that one's blood type influences the body's response to different foods, this guide aims to empower individuals to make informed choices that enhance their overall well-being.

The understanding of Blood Type A characteristics and the scientific insights into the genetic factors influencing dietary preferences form the foundation of this guide. By delving into the science behind Blood Type A, readers gain valuable knowledge about how their bodies process nutrients, fostering a deeper connection between dietary choices and personal health.

The importance of tailored nutrition to Blood Type A individuals is emphasized throughout the guide, highlighting the potential benefits of aligning one's diet with the specific needs of their blood type. From the selection of foods that complement Blood Type A characteristics to the creation of a Blood Type A-friendly kitchen, this guide serves as a practical resource for implementing sustainable dietary changes.

Examining the health implications associated with Blood Type A, the guide sheds light on how dietary choices can positively impact various aspects of well-being. By addressing the potential health benefits and promoting a balanced lifestyle, the guide encourages individuals to take charge of their health journey through mindful eating.

The cookbook section of the guide provides an extensive and elaborate list of Blood Type A-friendly foods, both to enjoy and to limit. From nutrient-rich ingredients to delicious recipes that cater specifically to Blood Type A requirements, the cookbook offers a diverse array of options, making the culinary experience enjoyable, satisfying, and health-conscious.

Furthermore, the 28-day meal plan provides a practical and structured approach to incorporating Blood Type A-friendly recipes into daily life. From breakfast to dinner, including snacks and desserts, the meal plan offers a variety of flavors and nutritional benefits, ensuring a well-rounded and satisfying dining experience.

In crafting a Blood Type A-friendly kitchen, the guide delves into the practical aspects of shopping and offers valuable tips for making informed choices at the grocery store. This, coupled with the detailed food lists, empowers readers to navigate the aisles confidently, ensuring that their pantry and refrigerator are stocked with wholesome and compatible options.

Ultimately, the Blood Type A Cookbook and Food List Guide serve as a holistic resource, blending scientific understanding with practical application. By embracing the tailored approach to nutrition outlined in this guide, individuals with Blood Type A can embark on a journey toward improved well-being, discovering the joys of delicious, health-conscious eating that complements their unique genetic makeup. Always consult with healthcare professionals or nutritionists for personalized advice, but armed with the knowledge from this guide, individuals can confidently navigate their dietary choices and embark on a path toward a healthier and more vibrant lifestyle.